HEY, LET'S TALK

BOYS PUBERTY

PARENT GUIDE

HELPING **YOU** LEAD YOUR PRETEEN THROUGH PUBERTY QUESTIONS, CONCERNS, AND REALITIES.

HEALTH
101

HEALTH 101 CURRICULUM

EMILY KISZKA, MA, BS, HEALTH EDUCATION

Published in the United States by: Health 101, LLC.

Content Production and Design: Emily Kiszka

Workbook ISBN (US): 979-8-89412-986-0

10 9 8 7 6 5 4 3 2 1
1st edition, 2024
Printed in the United States of America

Hi Parents-

Welcome to "Hey, Let's Talk- Puberty Workbook for Boys": A personalized learning experience centered around puberty and all of the life changes that preteens experience.

As the two of you journey through the "Hey, Let's Talk- Workbook for Boys," this parent guide will walk you through each page with overviews, pointers, and suggestions.

The main goal is to minimize awkwardness when it comes to these difficult conversations while increasing authentic communication and an overall self-confidence and sense of self in your preteen.

It's so great you're here!

Emily

Health Educator and Mom

" I loved how **COMFORTABLE** this workbook experience felt for my son and me. It felt like '*no big deal*' and '*nothing to feel embarrassed about,*' which is exactly what we needed."

EXAMPLE
of page layouts

PAGE FOUND
Corresponding page in student workbook.

BASIC OVERVIEW
Explains what's required in the activity.

PAGE 4
in student
workbook

This worksheet asks the participant to **draw 3 pictures of himself,** one as a young child, one of himself right now, and one that predicts how he sees himself in the future.

PARENT REFERENCE

OBJECTIVES

THE PURPOSE
Clarifies the goal of the activity.

while realizing that all changes happen slowly.

• This is setting the stage for the topic of puberty by giving the participant a chance to **notice change.**

THE TAKE AWAY
States the activity's main message and gives parent(s) the perfect thing to say.

MAIN CONCEPT

• **Parent says:** *"What are ways that your baby body changed into your child body?"* Discuss getting taller, stronger, faster.

EXAMPLE | KEY

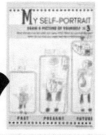

HEALTH

HEALTH

AN UPCLOSE GLIMPSE
Provides a visual of completed work and answer keys when necessary.

PAGE 1
in student
workbook

PRETEEN
CHECKS OFF
AS HE GOES

HEY, LET'S TALK!

CHECK IT OFF ✔

ICE
BREAKERS

PUBERTY
BASICS

CENTERING
REMINDERS

IN-DEPTH
CONTENT

SELF-
CONFIDENCE
WORK

ADDITIONAL
RESOURCES

HEAL

PARENT REFERENCES

PAGES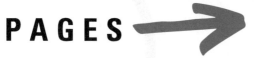

1-5

ICE BREAKERS

Welcome Letter, Introduce Yourself, My Self-Portrait, and More About Me

HEALTH
101

PARENT REFERENCE

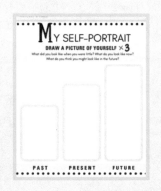

This worksheet asks the participant to **draw 3 pictures of himself,** one as a young child, one of himself right now, and one that predicts how he sees himself in the future.

OBJECTIVES

- This activity gives the participant a chance to **reflect** on his growth over his whole life while realizing that all changes happen slowly.

- This is setting the stage for the topic of puberty by giving the participant a chance to **notice change**.

MAIN CONCEPT

- Our bodies are always changing.

- Change happens slowly.

- **Parent says:** *"What are ways that your baby body changed into your child body?"* Discuss getting taller, stronger, faster.

EXAMPLE | KEY

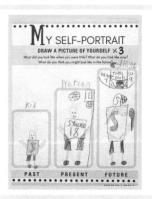

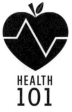

HEALTH
101

PAGE 5
in student
workbook

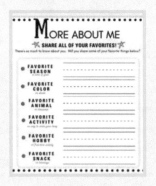

This worksheet asks the participant to write down some of his **favorite things**. This can be a quick activity or it can lead to comfortable and fun conversations. Maybe you can share responses for *your* favorite things as well.

OBJECTIVES

- Participant **identifies** things about himself.
- Noticing these things sets a foundation for **recognizing** that he has an inner-self, unrelated to his physical body. This includes his internal perspectives, opinions, and values.

MAIN CONCEPT

- We have an **"inside self."** It makes us who we are.
- Our "inside self" is special and valuable.
- **Parent says:** *"What else makes up who you are?"* Discuss: who he cares about and his passions, interests, values, and personality strengths.

EXAMPLE | KEY

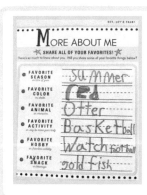

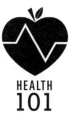

HEALTH
101

PARENT REFERENCE

PARENT REFERENCES

PAGES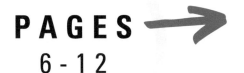
6-12

PUBERTY BASICS

Puberty Defined, Myth or Fact, Puberty Feelings, Whatcha Think? Straight Talk, and Puberty Maze

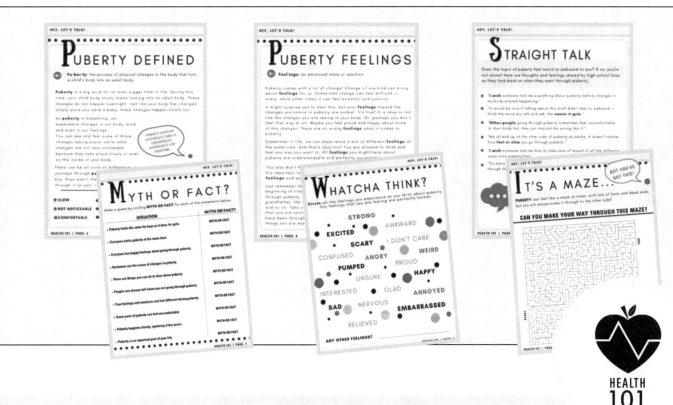

PARENT REFERENCE

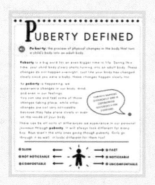

OBJECTIVES

MAIN CONCEPT

EXAMPLE | KEY

Here is where the topic of **Puberty** is introduced.

Read through this page together with the participant.

- Participant will **recognize** puberty as a time of change for his physical body– from child body to adult body.

- Participant will **understand** that puberty is normal and that it happens to everyone.

- Everyone goes through a time called **puberty** where the body slowly begins to physically change from a child body to an adult body.

- **Parent says:** *"Look at your pictures on page 4! It took a long time for your baby body to turn into a child body, right? Growing into your adult body will be slow, too."*

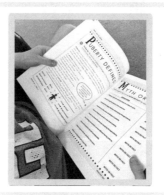

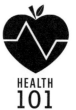

HEALTH
101

PARENT REFERENCE

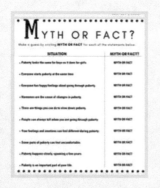

This is a pre-survey. Ask your child to try his best answering each statement. Read through the statements together if desired, but don't reveal the answers. You can mention that this is something you will look at together at the end.

OBJECTIVES

- Child reads or listens to statements and independently circles **MYTH or FACT** for each puberty statement.

MAIN CONCEPT

- This serves as **baseline data** for you, regarding what your child may know or not know.

- **Parent says:** *"Just try your best here. It does not matter if your answers are right or wrong. Take your best guess!"*

EXAMPLE | KEY

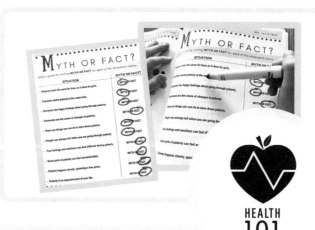

HEALTH
101

PARENT REFERENCE

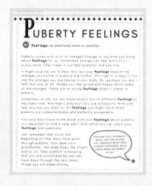

Here is where the topic of **feelings** surrounding puberty is introduced.

Read through this page together with the participant.

OBJECTIVES

- Participant will **recognize** that changes can bring about feelings. Not everyone has the same feelings about puberty.

- Participant will **understand** that all feelings are okay and that we never have to be alone with our feelings.

MAIN CONCEPT

- All feelings are valid. We never have to be alone in dealing with feelings.

- **Parent says:** *"Any feelings you are having about puberty are okay. We can even have more than one feeling at the same time! We can feel both nervous and curious or excited and awkward. You can always share your feelings with me."*

EXAMPLE | KEY

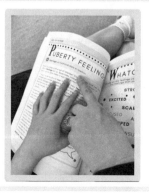

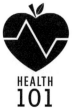

HEALTH
101

PARENT REFERENCE

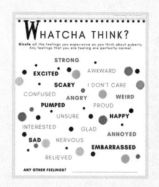

Here is where **feelings** are personalized. Participant will circle any feelings that resonate with him. He can circle as many as he wants.

OBJECTIVES

- Participant will circle all feelings that resonate with him.

MAIN CONCEPT

- We experience a lot of feelings in life, especially during puberty. Recognizing them is important.
- **Optional parent comments:** *"That makes sense," "I totally get that," "I know. It can definitely feel like that," "It's so great that you notice your feelings," "These feelings can change each day."*

EXAMPLE | KEY

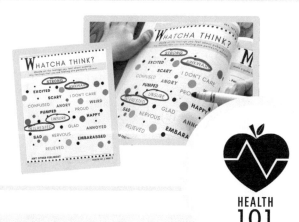

HEALTH
101

PAGES
10 + 11
in student
workbook

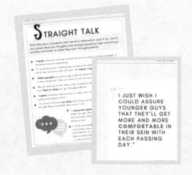

These pages contain quotes from **real-life** high school boys sharing their perspectives having already gone through puberty.

Read through and share your own thoughts or feelings, if you wish.

OBJECTIVES

- Participant will **realize** that older peers have been through this too and will potentially feel a sense of encouragement or camaraderie.

MAIN CONCEPT

- Older boys have been through this time of puberty too, even dads, uncles, and grandpas; and they survived!

- **Parent says:** *"Were there any quotes here that stood out to you? Were there any that you feel too?"*

EXAMPLE | KEY

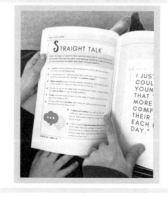

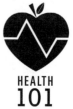

HEALTH
101

PARENT REFERENCE

PARENT REFERENCE

PAGE 12
in student
workbook

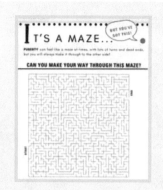

This worksheet is an optional activity if your child likes a little challenge! Using a pencil, he needs to start on the left side starting point and work his way through to the end.

OBJECTIVES

- Participant will complete the maze, even if that means trying several times!

MAIN CONCEPT

- Puberty can feel a lot like a maze: no direction, confusing paths, and wrong turns.

- **Parent says:** *"There is always a way through. It might take some patience with the process, but you will always make it through to the other side."*

EXAMPLE | KEY

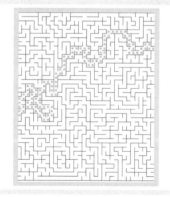

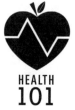

HEALTH
101

PARENT REFERENCES

PAGES
13-19

→

CENTERING REMINDERS

It's Still You, Heart Qualities, Fist Bump, Make a Plane, and Mystery Message

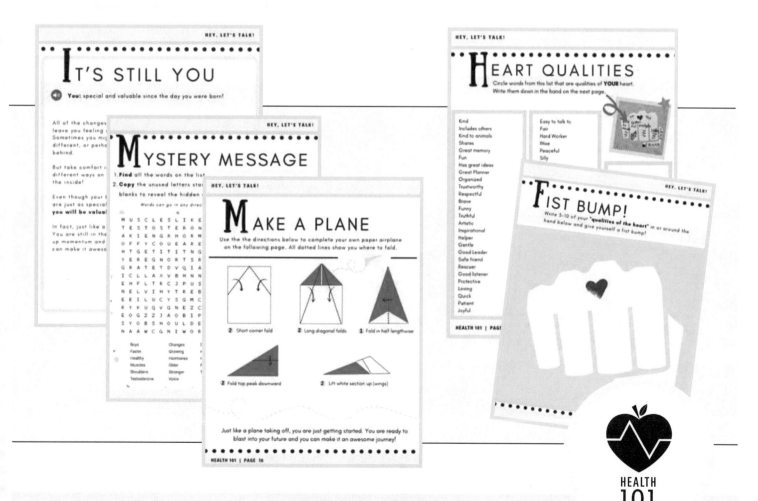

PAGE 13
in student
workbook

PARENT REFERENCE

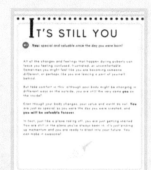

Here is where the concept of **"inner self"** is explored in greater depth. Read through this page together with your child.

OBJECTIVES

- Participant will **recognize** that his inner self does not change, even though his outer self is changing.

- Participant will begin to **develop** an awareness of his inherent value and worth.

MAIN CONCEPT

- Even though his body changes, it's still the same person on the inside.

- His body may change but his value and "specialness" do not.

- **Parent says,** *"You are special because you are you! You have been special since the day you were born and you'll be special forever."*

EXAMPLE | KEY

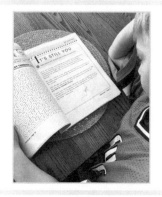

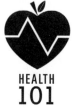

HEALTH
101

PARENT REFERENCE

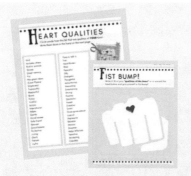

Participant will explore what makes him special. First, he will circle all of the qualities and traits he feels apply to him on **page 14**. Then, he will write some or all of the traits in or around the fist on **page 15**.

OBJECTIVES

- Participant will **review** a list of **"heart qualities"** and identify what qualities he sees in himself.

- Participant will **display** his heart qualities on or around the fist (**pg. 15**).

- Participant can even give his fist a **fist bump (pg. 15)**!

MAIN CONCEPT

- Your heart is good and it's made up of unique **"heart qualities"** that belong to you. They make you interesting and unique.

- **Parent says:** *"Even though we see changes in life and in our bodies, your "Heart Qualities" can stay the same. You can even add more "Heart Qualities" to your life as you grow!"*

EXAMPLE | KEY

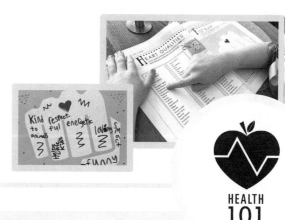

**HEALTH
101**

PAGES
16-19
in student
workbook

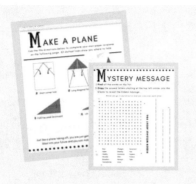

- Participant will create a paper airplane using the directions (page 16) and the blank page (page 17).

- Participant will complete a **word search** and decode the **mystery message** (page 19).

OBJECTIVES

- These pages are optional activities that give participant a chance to have fun while he **reflects** on his value, even in the midst of change.

MAIN CONCEPT

- This time does not change him, but adds even more strength and uniqueness to who he is.

EXAMPLE | KEY

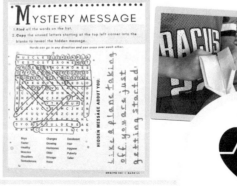

HEALTH
101

PARENT REFERENCES

PAGES → **IN-DEPTH CONTENT**

20-51

Word Identification, Word Search, Questions, Hmmm.., Identification, Let's Talk, Rate Your Understanding, and Myth or Fact

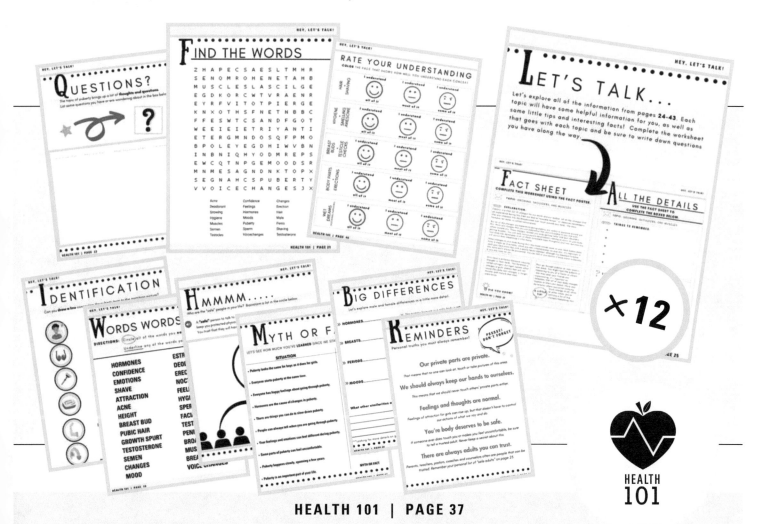

HEALTH
101

PARENT REFERENCE

Participant will get familiar with words that are associated with puberty. On **page 20**, he will **circle** the words he is familiar with and **underline** words that he is not familiar with. He can gain further familiarity by completing a word search on **page 21**, if he'd like.

OBJECTIVES

- Participant will **identify** what words he knows and what words he does not know.
- Participant will **familiarize** himself with all words associated with puberty.

MAIN CONCEPT

- It's important to get acquainted with all of the new words surrounding puberty.
- **Parent says:** *"Have you heard of some of these words? We'll be exploring all of them in this workbook together so that you feel comfortable knowing what all of them mean."*

EXAMPLE | KEY

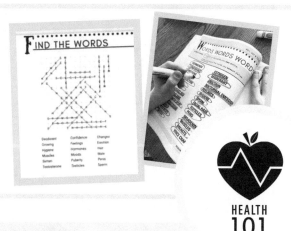

HEALTH
101

PAGE 22
in student
workbook

PARENT REFERENCE

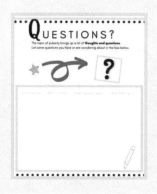

Before beginning puberty content, participant can list questions he has. He can ask anything he is wondering about—concerning anything!

OBJECTIVES

- Participant will identify any questions he has moving into the following workbook pages of puberty content.

MAIN CONCEPT

- **Parent says:** *"You don't have to write them out in sentences. You can just jot down words or thoughts, if that's easier for you."*
- ***Parent note:*** Give your child space to do this part on his own. Also, if your child feels uncomfortable with this, or claims to have no questions, he **doesn't have to** do this part.

EXAMPLE | KEY

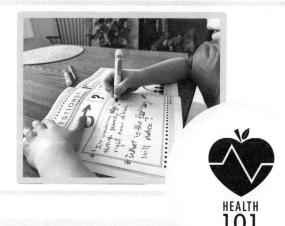

HEALTH
101

PAGE **23**
in student
workbook

PARENT REFERENCE

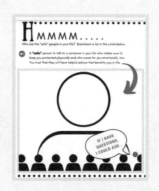

Participant will be introduced to the concept of a "safe" person, and he will create a list (even if short) of the safe people in his life that he can bring his questions to as they arise.

OBJECTIVES

- Participant will **read** and define what a "safe" person is.

- Participant will **brainstorm** a list of "safe" people in his life that he can always bring his questions to.

MAIN CONCEPT

- We must know who our "safe" people are when we have questions.

- **Parent says:** *"We will ALWAYS have questions about our bodies and about life. Even adults have questions! It's important to remember safe and trustworthy people to whom we can go with our questions."*

EXAMPLE | KEY

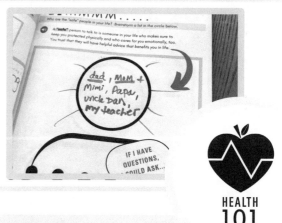

HEALTH 101

PAGE 24
in student
workbook

PARENT REFERENCE

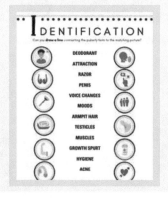

Participant will take word identification a step further through matching the puberty term to the correct picture.

OBJECTIVES

- Participant will **match** the puberty term to the correct picture.

MAIN CONCEPT

- Participant will grow increasingly comfortable with puberty terms and concepts through simply noticing terms and their connections to images.

EXAMPLE | KEY

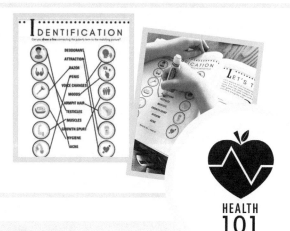

HEALTH
101

Let's talk...

This section of the workbook will dive into puberty content. Encourage your child to write on the corresponding **"All the Details"** worksheets as he navigates through each topic. Doing so will give him the chance to **reflect** and **check-in** about things he has learned and things he still wonders about.

Feelings, Growing, Hygiene, Hair, Shaving, Body Parts and Changes, Erections, Attraction, Voice Changes

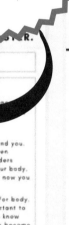

Information organized by topic!

Fact Sheet

COMPLETE THIS WORKSHEET USING THE FACT POSTER.

✉ **TOPIC:** GROWING, SHOULDERS, AND MUSCLES

📖 **EXPLANATION**

Puberty is a time full of changes for our minds and our bodies. The changes we experience during this time are due to "invisible forces," or hormones, that are released into the bloodstream and travel around your body. The hormone for males is called testosterone.

Not all of the changes you experience during puberty are visible to everyone around you. But, there are changes that you will experience that are noticeable to you and even others around you. These changes include your body getting taller and your shoulders getting broader. You will even notice muscle development starting to occur on your body. Your body has developed in all of these noticeable ways throughout your life, but now you will notice them happening a little faster.

Other changes in your body during this time could include acne on your face and/or body. Acne is made up of pimples, which are red, irritated bumps on your skin. It's important to wash your face every day with a gentle facial cleanser, although it's important to know that acne can't always be prevented. You can talk to your doctor if acne starts to become a very big issue for you.

Girls have a different hormone causing changes in their body. This hormone is called estrogen. Estrogen causes other changes in girls' bodies that will not cause the same fast changes in height, muscle, and stature that boys experience.

Boys go through puberty at their body's own pace. You might feel like puberty is happening to you at a faster or slower rate than what your friends are experiencing. It's important to remember that all of your body changes happen at their own speed. There may be seasons where you're not noticing much change at all while at other times, you're noticing a lot of big changes happening fast.

💡 **DID YOU KNOW?**

💬 **A LITTLE TIP!**

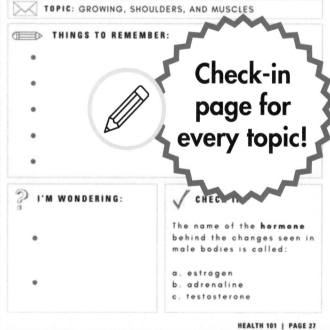

All The Details

USE THE FACT SHEET TO COMPLETE THE BOXES BELOW.

✉ **TOPIC:** GROWING, SHOULDERS, AND MUSCLES

📖 **THINGS TO REMEMBER:**

-
-
-
-

Check-in page for every topic!

❓ **I'M WONDERING:**

✓ **CHECK-IN**

The name of the **hormone** behind the changes seen in male bodies is called:

a. estrogen
b. adrenaline
c. testosterone

PARENT REFERENCE

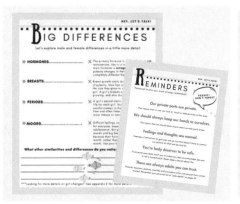

As a follow-up to page 46 in the workbook, these pages highlight key differences between male and female bodies while encouraging safety and respect.

OBJECTIVES

- Participant will **read** through the differences girls experience during puberty and beyond. They can record any remaining questions they may have.

- **Appendix E** will be helpful while on this page.

MAIN CONCEPT

- Girls' and boys' bodies are **different** and puberty creates even more differences.

- **Important note:** Boys often witness changes in girls before they experience changes in their own bodies. Girls can begin experiencing puberty changes as early as third grade.

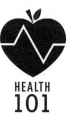

HEALTH
101

PAGE 50
in student
workbook

PARENT REFERENCE

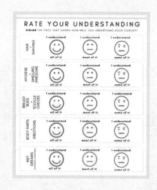

Participant **shades in** one face in each row that reflects his level of understanding regarding the puberty topics covered in pages **26-47**.

OBJECTIVES

- Participant **reflects** on how comfortable he feels in his knowledge of each of the puberty topics covered on **pages 26-47**.

MAIN CONCEPT

- Parent can **assess** any areas of confusion regarding the puberty topics that were covered in **pages 26-47**.

EXAMPLE | KEY

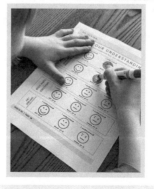

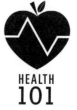

HEALTH
101

PAGE 51
in student
workbook

PARENT REFERENCE

Participant completes the same worksheet as he did on **page 7**. This time, he should demonstrate more of an understanding of puberty topics. Review together, after participant is finished.

OBJECTIVES

- Participant reads or listens to statements and independently circles **MYTH or FACT** for each puberty statement.

- Parent and participant review answers together.

MAIN CONCEPT

- This serves as **summative data** for you, regarding what your child now knows or does not know.

- **Parent says:** *"Now that you've covered all of the puberty topics, let's see if you answer these statements about puberty any differently than you did in the beginning."*

EXAMPLE | KEY

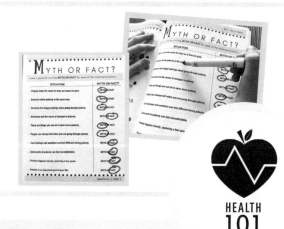

HEALTH
101

PARENT REFERENCES

PAGES 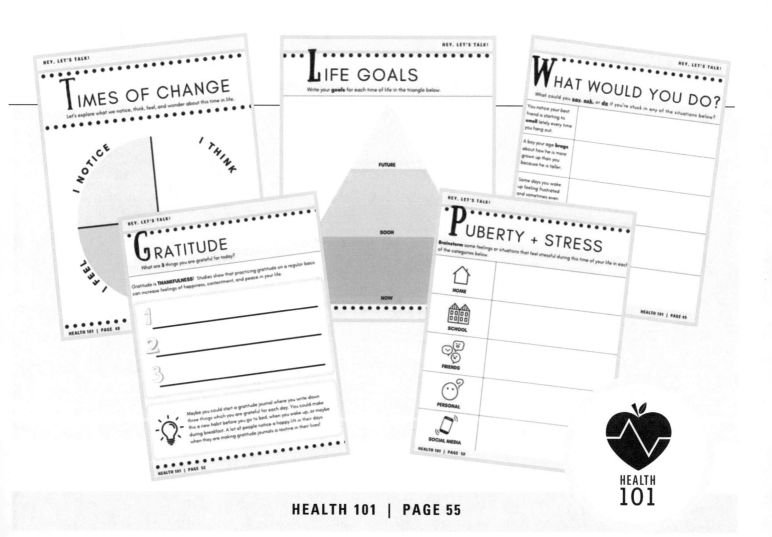 **SELF-CONFIDENCE WORK**

52-56

Times of Change, What Would You Do?, Puberty + Stress, Life Goals, and Gratitude

PARENT REFERENCE

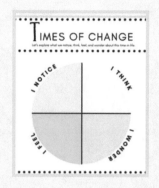

Participant **records** anything in his life that he notices, thinks, feels, and/or wonders during this time in his life. These can be positive, negative, or anything in between.

OBJECTIVES

- Participant **identifies** things in his life that he notices, thinks, feels, and/or wonders.

MAIN CONCEPT

- **Noticing** these things and putting them into words can be helpful in decreasing stress, minimizing anxiety, and making personal realities easier to talk about.
- **Parent says:** *"This time is a very unique time in your life. You probably have a lot of random things you notice, think, feel, and wonder."*

EXAMPLE | KEY

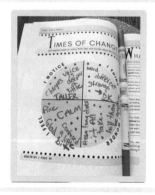

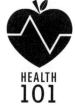

**HEALTH
101**

PAGE 53
in student
workbook

Participant **responds** to each hypothetical situation regarding what he could do.

OBJECTIVES

- Participant **problem solves** through the presentation of realistic situations.

MAIN CONCEPT

- Confusing and shocking situations can come up a lot during puberty. It's important to work through ways we can get through them.
- **Parent says:** *"We can work through these situations together so you feel more prepared if they ever happen."*

EXAMPLE | KEY

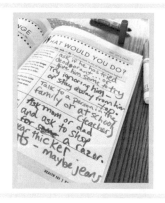

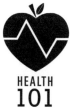

HEALTH
101

PAGE 54
in student
workbook

PARENT REFERENCE

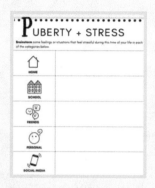

Participant lists sources of stress in any or all areas of life. Parent can get a bird's-eye view of each area of life that may require extra attention or care.

OBJECTIVES

• Participant recognizes and shares aspects of life that feel stressful.

MAIN CONCEPT

• Recognizing areas of stress is important so the participant can process his feelings and reach out for help.

• **Parent says:** *"This is an activity that you can do over and over again. Any time you're overwhelmed, you can make a stress list. Some people call this a 'brain dump'."*

EXAMPLE | KEY

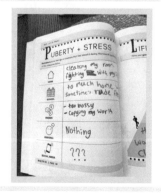

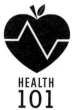

HEALTH
101

PAGE 55
in student
workbook

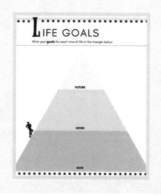

Participant sets some **life goals** for today and his future.

OBJECTIVES

- Participant creates a **vision** for his life.
- Participant **records** big and small goals.

MAIN CONCEPT

- Goal setting is important in fostering a healthy confidence in boys. It helps take their minds off the "here and now" by opening their eyes to all the possibilities the future holds.
- **Parent says:** *"When you feel overwhelmed, it helps to look ahead. You can create your future to look any way you want it to!"*

EXAMPLE | KEY

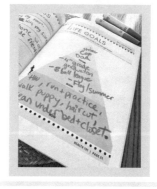

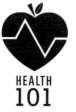

HEALTH
101

PARENT REFERENCE

PARENT REFERENCE

Gratitude is a powerful tool in achieving happiness. Here, the participant will construct a list of three things he is thankful for. He should be encouraged to continue this practice daily or weekly.

OBJECTIVES

- Participant writes three things he is grateful for.
- Participant is introduced to the fact that practicing gratitude increases overall happiness and contentment.

MAIN CONCEPT

- Participant focuses on positive things in his life- both big and small.
- **Parent says:** *"Your grateful list doesn't always have to be big things. It can list the small things too- things we often overlook or take for granted, like clean drinking water."*

EXAMPLE | KEY

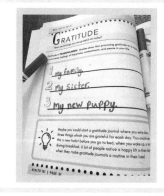

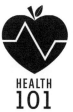

HEALTH
101

PARENT REFERENCES

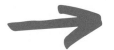

ADDITIONAL RESOURCES

Anonymous Questions, Journal Paper, Appendix Images A-F, and Glossary.

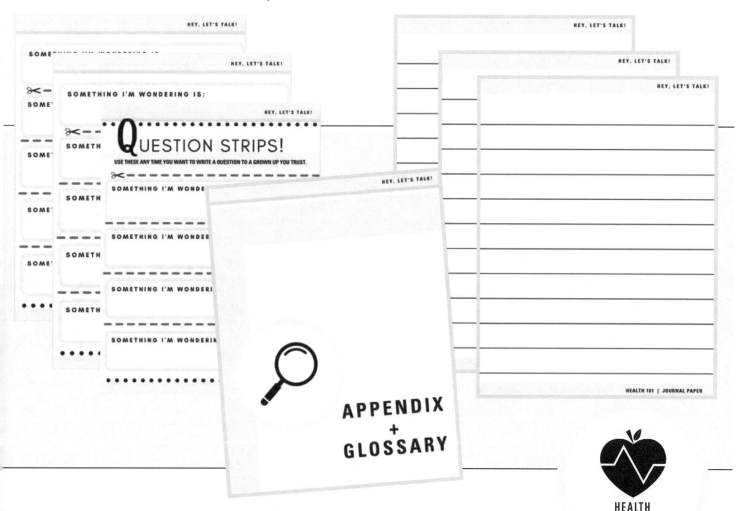

PARENT REFERENCE

This template is an optional resource for you and your child to use to enhance communication with each other when it comes to tough questions and answers.

OBJECTIVES

- Parent and child can communicate using these "Anonymous Question" paper strips as necessary.
- Anonymous Question paper strips can be located in your child's workbook.

MAIN CONCEPT

- Sometimes these topics can be uncomfortable- especially for kids. These are available for your child in case he feels more comfortable asking you something in writing.

EXAMPLE | KEY

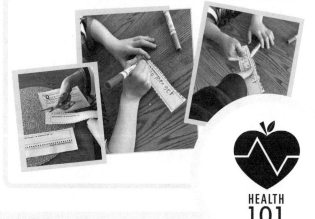

HEALTH
101

PARENT REFERENCE

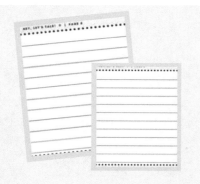

JOURNAL PAPER
in student workbook

Participant can use this free space for notes or journaling, if desired.

OBJECTIVES

- Participant can reflect, dream, and share in this space.

MAIN CONCEPT

- These pages can be used as extra space for reflection on puberty, feelings, and experiences.

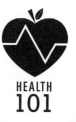

HEALTH
101

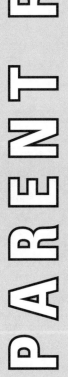

PARENT REFERENCE

Participant can reference the Appendix as he completes the workbook.

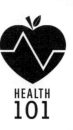

OBJECTIVES

- Participant uses these pages for more details as needed. They are found in the back of the workbook.

HEALTH
101

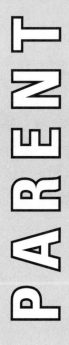

GLOSSARY

in student workbook

Participant can reference the Glossary as he completes the workbook.

OBJECTIVES

- Participant uses these pages for more details as needed. They are found in the back of the workbook.

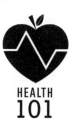

HEALTH
101

APPENDIX
+
GLOSSARY

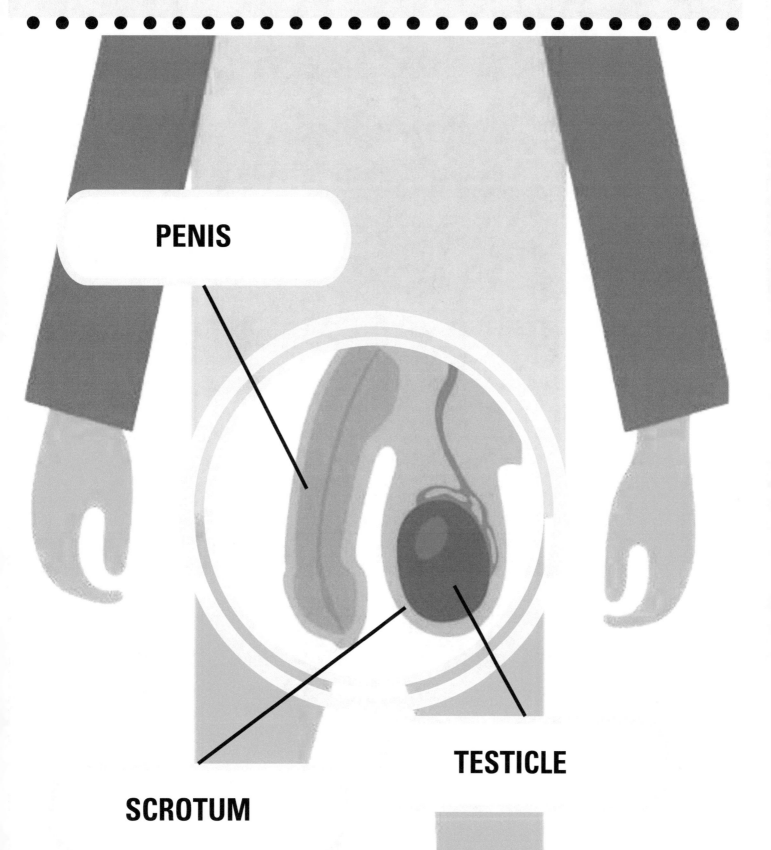

PENIS

SCROTUM

TESTICLE

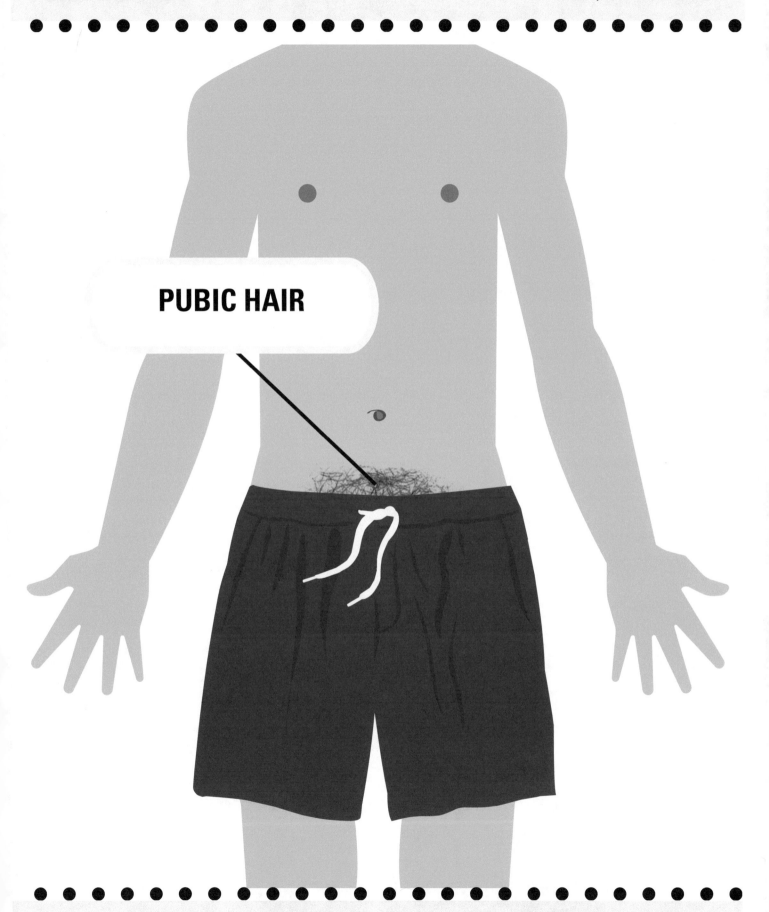

PUBIC HAIR

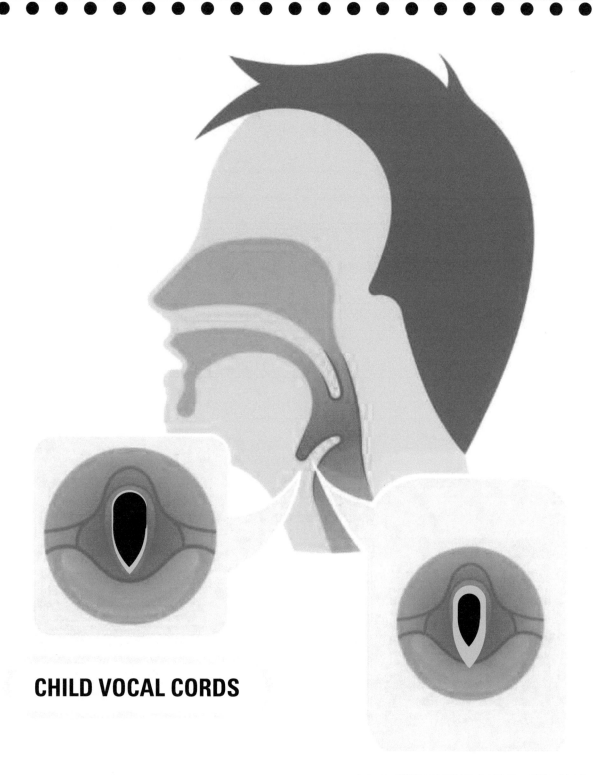

CHILD VOCAL CORDS

MATURE VOCAL CORDS

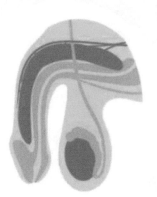

NO ERECTION

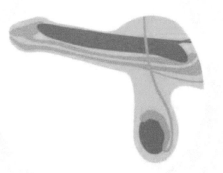

ERECTION

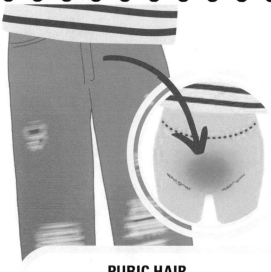

PUBIC HAIR

Girls get pubic hair in the same "pubic region," just as you do.

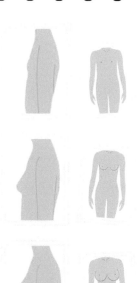

BREASTS

Breasts come in all shapes and sizes and begin developing for girls at different times over the course of puberty.

Girls start wearing bras to help support this area of their body which gives them more support.

GIRL DIFFERENCES

Girls' bodies are very different from boys' bodies. Those changes become even greater during puberty and into adulthood. Here are a few glimpses of some existing differences:

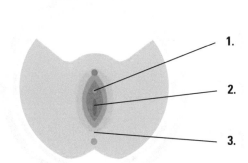

1.
2.
3.

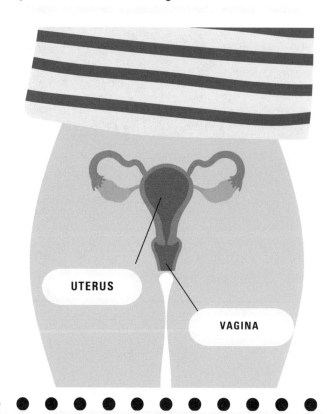

UTERUS

VAGINA

1. **The Urethra**
The urethra is where urine (pee) leaves the body.

2. **The Vagina**
The vagina is where blood leaves the body during the period and it is where the baby leaves the body during childbirth.

3. **The Anus**
The anus is where feces (poop) leaves the body.

SHOWER
EVERY DAY

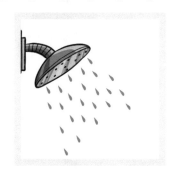

Shower or bathe every day!
Use soap everywhere, but especially in all of the cracks or crevices of your body. It's also important to completely dry off, especially in all of those places (butt crack, arm pits, toes, etc). And be sure to hang your towel up in order to dry it properly so that bacteria and smells cannot grow on it.

DON'T FORGET!

In order to **smell awesome**, we have to do certain things.
And we have to do those things more often during puberty and beyond.

DEODORANT
EVERY DAY

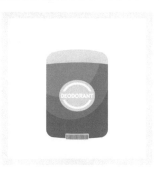

Wear deodorant every day!
You may not smell in the mornin or right after a shower, but rubbing deodorant in your armpits before odors start is very important in order to make sure you don't smell all day. Wear it every day!

ORAL CARE
2X / DAY

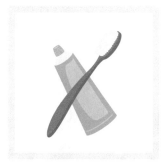

Brush your teeth twice a day!
In fact, your mouth needs more than that! Don't forget mouthwash, floss, and tongue scrapers. Those three things help to minimize bad breath. And remember, you won't always know your breath smells- but others will! So keep up with all of these things!

LAUNDRY
AS NEEDED

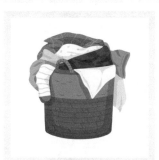

Wash your clothes!
Even if you wash your body and have great oral care, others might still think you smell if you aren't washing your clothes enough. Throw your clothes in the laundry after wearing them, even if they aren't stained, sweaty, or dirty!

ACNE: Skin issues and irritations comprised of blackheads, whiteheads, and red pimples (or zits) that can surface on the face and also other areas of the body.

ADOLESCENCE: A time period where a young person goes through a process of developing from a child into an adult.

ATTRACTION: Feelings of interest in a person's looks, personality and/or actions. Desiring to be closer to that person.

BREAST: A protuberance or rounded bump or mass, surmounted by a nipple, located on each side of the upper chest of a woman. Begins as a breast bud during puberty. Also commonly known as "boobs."

BREAST BUD: A tiny mass under the nipple that is the beginning stage of breast development. Can be painful at times.

ERECTION: An enlarged and hard/ridged state of the penis.

ESTROGEN: A naturally-occurring hormone that regulates development and body function in females.

GENITALS: For males, includes the penis and testicles. For females, includes the vagina and skin outside surrounding the urethra and vagina.

GROWTH SPURT: A period when a child's body rapidly grows in height and stature.

HORMONES: Chemical substances that are secreted by the body internally into the bloodstream.

HYGIENE: Keeping the body and its surroundings clean to promote health.

PENIS: External male genitalia. Contains the urethra that carries urine (pee) and semen and sperm out of the body.

PRETEEN: A young person who is not yet a teenager; usually between the ages of 11-13.

PUBERTY: A time of life where a child's body begins to change into an adult's body.

PUBIC HAIR: Coarse, dark hair that grows on the pubic region during and after puberty.

SCROTUM: A sack made of skin tissue found on the outside of a male's body between the penis and anus.

TESTICLES: Two egg-shaped glands inside the scrotum that produce sperm and male hormones.

TESTOSTERONE: The naturally-occurring hormone that regulates development in males.

VOCAL CORDS: Folds of tissue in the throat that vibrate when speaking to create the voice.

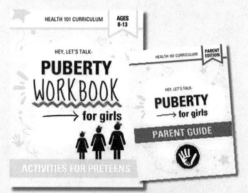

Equipping parents, informing kids- taking the **awkward** out of PUBERTY talks!

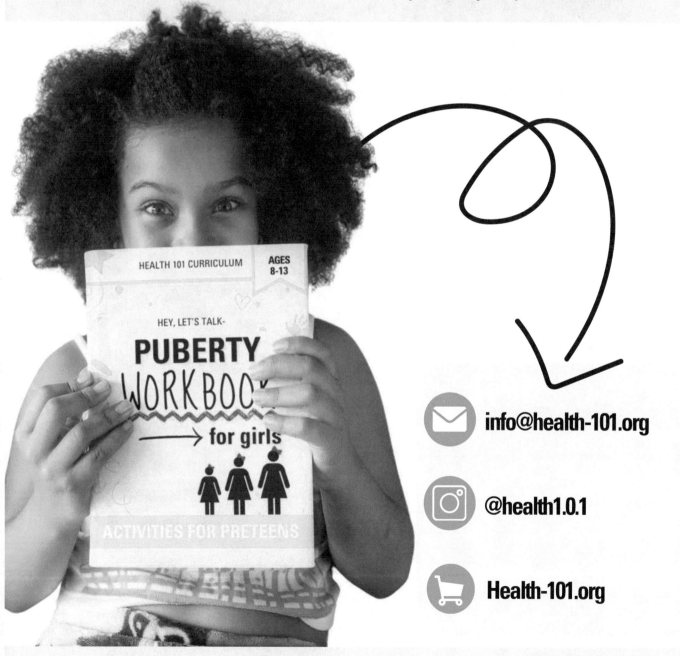

info@health-101.org

@health1.0.1

Health-101.org

HEALTH 101, LLC.

Made in United States
Troutdale, OR
08/03/2024

21758231R00055